Yoga For Weight Loss

Yoga Weight Loss Secrets to
Melt Fat, Trim Inches and
Get a Youthful Sexy Body—FAST!

Olivia Summers

Published in The USA by:
Success Life Publishing
125 Thomas Burke Dr.
Hillsborough, NC 27278

Copyright © 2015 by Olivia Summers

ISBN-10: 151168271X

ALL RIGHTS RESERVED. No part of this publication may be reproduced or transmitted in any form whatsoever, electronic, or mechanical, including photocopying, recording, or by any informational storage or retrieval system without the express written permission from the author, except for the use of brief quotations in a book review.

Disclaimer:

Every effort has been made to accurately represent this book and its potential. Results vary with every individual, and your results may or may not be different from those depicted. No promises, guarantees or warranties, whether stated or implied, have been made that you will produce any specific result from this book. Your efforts are individual and unique, and may vary from those shown. Your success depends on your efforts, background and motivation.

The material in this publication is provided for educational and informational purposes only and is not intended as medical advice. The information contained in this book should not be used to diagnose or treat any illness, metabolic disorder, disease or health problem. Always consult your physician or health care provider before beginning any nutrition or exercise program. Use of the programs, advice, and information contained in this book is at the sole choice and risk of the reader.

Table of Contents

Introduction 1
Chapter 1: Yoga 101 3
Chapter 2: Why Yoga for Weight Loss? 8
Chapter 3: 15 Yoga Poses for Weight Loss 15
Tree Pose 15
Chair Pose 17
High Lunge Pose 19
Intense Side Stretch Pose 21
Downward Facing Dog 23
Cobra Pose 25
Warrior I Pose 27
Fish Pose 29
Upward Facing Dog 31
Boat Pose 33
Chaturanga Pose (Four Limbed Staff) 35
Bow Pose 36
Supported Shoulder Stand 38
Side Plank Pose 41
Handstand 43
Chapter 4: Yoga, Food and You 49
Chapter 5: Mindful Eating 60
Chapter 6: Developing Healthy Habits to Lose Weight Faster 69
Conclusion 74

Introduction

Thank you so much for purchasing my book "Yoga For Weight Loss." My name is Olivia Summers and I'm a Certified Yoga Teacher and in this book I'm going to share with you some of the **best secrets** of losing weight through yoga.

The framework of this book is based on my 13+ years of experience in the practice of yoga and what has helped guide me along the way. It may be hard to believe, but I actually used to be more than 50 pounds overweight.

Did yoga magically transform me and help me drop those 50 pounds overnight? Absolutely not. But I can honestly say yoga has been the catalyst for my new healthy lifestyle and my dramatic weight loss results. And I know that yoga can help you as well!

Is it going to be easy and without hard work? No, you're going to have to truly want to change and make the commitment to do so, but I know that yoga can help get you there.

I hope that the tips and advice I've compiled in this book help you to have a better understanding of how yoga can help you accomplish your weight loss goals and point you in the direction of a healthier lifestyle overall.

I know that if you follow and apply my advice to your life then you can have the same healthy and life changing results that I've gotten from yoga.

Chapter 1: Yoga 101

A Brief History of Yoga

Traditionally speaking, the term yoga actually comes from the Sanskrit root word 'yuj'—which means "to yoke or harness." How does this relate to yoga? Well, in India, in order to control an ox you would have to harness it to a wagon. This is basically a metaphor for yoga—you use it as a way to train and unite your body, mind and spirit.

A lot of people think yoga is a form of religion, but it is actually a philosophy that came into practice in India over 5,000 years ago! Although it is sometimes *part* of practicing Buddhism and Hinduism, yoga in and of itself is not a religion. Oh and just a fun fact for you: did you know that there have been images discovered from ancient Egypt over 5,000+ years ago that depict Egyptians in Tree poses and other asanas? Pretty cool!

The founding father of ashtanga yoga (or the Eight Limbs of Yoga) and author of the *Yoga Sutras* was Patanjali. Unfortunately, very little is known about who he was or where he came from—or even when exactly he lived. One thing is certain, though—if Patanjali had not completed his *Yoga Sutras* we probably wouldn't know much, if anything, about the yoga we practice today.

Patanjali's *Sutras* were a collection of 195 different philosophies about the practice of yoga. His book also outlined the eight individual "limbs" or types of yoga—asana (postures) being the most popular in Western culture.

In the late 19th and early 20th centuries many of the yoga gurus from India introduced yoga as a practice to Western civilization. However, it wasn't until around the 1980's that yoga became a more popular form of physical exercise in the Western world.

It's true that over the course of its lifetime yoga has taken on many different forms—when it started out it was much more about inward reflection and learning to just sit and be still. Now, however, our society's needs have changed and grown. Yoga has become much more of an exercise and a way to showcase our physical abilities.

Many "serious" yoga practitioners and gurus frown upon our commercialized version of yoga in the Western world. The reason for this is because they believe that yoga is meant to be much more than just exercise. Its traditional roots are founded in meditative and spiritual upbringing—becoming in tune to oneself in the process.

I agree with these gurus and in my personal practice I use yoga for spiritual and meditative purposes as well. However, yoga is something different for everyone and I don't think there's anything wrong with that. If you want to use yoga as a tool to lose weight then I think that it would be incredibly beneficial—it's all about what you make it and it's okay for that to look different for different people.

Most Popular Forms of Yoga

Aerial—Basically this is yoga...in a hammock! Aerial yoga was introduced in New York and is one of the newest forms of yoga. If you're the adventurous type and already have the more run-of-the-mill yoga classes under your belt then it might be time for you to give this a try.

Ashtanga—This is one of the oldest forms of yoga (remember Patanjali's *Sutras*?) and what we'll be using throughout this book. Ashtanga is made up of six different series' of postures and is used prevalently throughout the West.

Bikram—Bikram yoga was introduced and made popular in the 1970's. Most people looking to lose weight and torch calories during a yoga session turn to Bikram yoga. It's also known as "hot" yoga—and for good reason. The classes are 90 minutes long and consist of a series of 26 poses that are repeated twice during the session. The catch? The room is heated to 104F and a humidity of 40%!

Hatha—Hatha yoga is what all other types of yoga are founded on and uses a more holistic approach than newer variations of yoga. It is a combination of meditation, purification, breathing and postures. It is very gentle and is great for beginners.

Kundalini—This can be one of the most fun forms of yoga, in my opinion. Kundalini yoga is founded on the belief that there is latent energy coiled at the base of our spines and it needs to be released. Kundalini yoga uses meditation and breathing to activate your chakras and release built up energy.

Restorative—This one is pretty self-explanatory. This type of yoga is focused on using different props to restore your physical body with your mental state. It's a very gentle and relaxing form of yoga. It is especially beneficial to those who need to learn to slow down and relieve stress.

Vinyasa—The term Vinyasa originates from the Sanskrit language and actually means "breath-synchronized movement." Which is exactly what you're doing during this type of yoga. You move through a series of poses while at the same time using your exhaling and inhaling breaths to "dance" your way through each pose. It is also sometimes referred to as Vinyasa Flow.

These are just a few of the more popular types of yoga practiced today in Western culture. The types of yoga best utilized for weight loss stem from these more popular versions of modern yoga, which we will cover in the next chapter.

Chapter 2: Yoga for Weight Loss

How Yoga Can Help You Lose Weight

In the previous chapter I outlined some of the most popular types of yoga. Logically, you might be asking yourself, 'What is the best type of yoga that will help me lose the most weight?' My answer: the type of yoga that you will actually do on a consistent basis.

As with any new diet or exercise program, it's easy to get caught up in all the details and trying to learn everything and making sure everything's just right. Sometimes we get so busy doing all this that it distracts us from the most important thing: doing! You have to take action to get anywhere, so find the type of yoga that speaks to you and your body and makes you want to come back and practice day after day.

With all that said, however, there are certain poses and types of yoga that are better for weight loss than others.

Best Types of Yoga to Lose Weight

Vinyasa Flow—If you try Vinyasa Flow as your weight loss yoga practice of choice, then expect to feel some burning muscles. Vinyasa yoga focuses on changing things up and keeping your body moving at a quick pace to give you an intense burn. These types of classes are often one of the liveliest types of yoga and if you hate the mundane and repetitive nature of other forms of yoga then you might prefer Vinyasa since no two classes are going to be the same.

You can expect to burn around 600 calories per hour.

PowerYoga—This is actually a type of Vinyasa yoga, but it goes at a much faster pace. The intent of this type of yoga is to maximize calorie burn while strengthening muscles to get an overall challenging workout in. This is also a more interpretive style of yoga so each teacher will probably have his or her own variation on the practice and as such, the style can change quite a bit from class to class.

You can expect to burn around 500 calories per hour doing PowerYoga.

Bikram Yoga—As I mentioned previously, Bikram yoga makes you sweat! This means good news for weight loss and it also provides a cleansing effect on the body. The 26 more traditional hatha poses are designed to address each function of all your bodily systems to help re-oxygenate and invigorate all the different parts of your body.

You can expect to burn around 500 calories per hour doing Bikram yoga.

What About Yoga for Relaxation?

Just because I didn't include the more calming forms of yoga on my list (like Hatha, Restorative and Ashtanga)—it doesn't mean that there isn't a place in your weight loss journey to practice these types of yoga.

I actually believe that restorative and relaxation yoga both provide immeasurable benefits and can help aid in weight loss tremendously.

I wouldn't personally recommend restorative or relaxation yoga to be your sole forms of practice if you're trying to lose weight, but they are great to supplement with the more intense yoga workouts.

My suggestion would be to do your more intense and cardio-type yoga workouts in the mornings or early afternoon to start your day and give you energy. Then, 2-3 evenings a week you could do a restorative or relaxation yoga class for stress relief.

This would help ease sore muscles and also help improve your flexibility at a much faster rate. Not to mention, if you do it in the evenings at home before bedtime it puts you in a better state of mind to fall asleep more peacefully.

Restorative yoga can be especially great for people who tend to have trouble sleeping because it forces you to focus on being still and quieting your mind. When you spend 30 minutes to an hour basically meditating you're going to increase your ability to be more restful and at peace while sleeping as well.

Yoga and Stress Relief

By practicing the restorative and relaxing forms of yoga you will also decrease your stress and tension levels by lowering your blood pressure and reducing your cortisol levels while all at the same time increasing your flexibility and strength.

Did you know that regular practice of yoga can actually re-program the way you react to stress? It's true. When you have to learn new poses in yoga class it can be a stressor in your mind—you learn to respond to the physical demands of stress on your body with steady breathing and mindfulness. Because of this your nervous system is going to learn to respond differently to stress over time and what you learn through yoga poses will also be carried over into other areas of your life that you may find stressful.

This won't come naturally, and at first you'll really have to focus on thinking positive thoughts and staying in control of your breathing. With enough practice, though, you will have programmed a new automatic response inside of your nervous system that helps you deal with stress day in and day out.

Maybe you're not so impressed with this new revelation. After all, stress isn't all that bad, is it? I mean, yes, it's annoying, but does it really hurt anything? Isn't it natural? Well, let's take a look...

Why is Stress Bad?

- *Causes disease—*
  Did you know that chronic stress can lead to the development of certain health problems like diabetes, heart disease, depression/anxiety, Alzheimer's and even death?
- *Ruins your teeth—*
  When you're stressed out you tend to grind your teeth, which can lead to tooth pain, jaw tightness and even gum disease.
- *Weakens your immune system—*
  When you're stressed out your immune system's defenses are going to be considerably lower, making you

much more susceptible to catching colds and infections. Yuck!

- *Accelerated aging—*
  When you're under a lot of stress you're actually preventing your cells from growing as quickly as they would under normal circumstances, which in turn leads to weak muscles, bad eyesight and even wrinkles!
- *Weight gain—*
  When we're stressed we tend to eat 40% more food than we would otherwise consume, which adds up to a lot of extra calories. If you're constantly stressed you could be overeating quite a bit –and packing on the pounds as well.

Are you convinced now? I hope that I've illustrated just how important it is to banish stress from your life—not only for your overall health, but especially if you have weight loss goals you want to achieve.

Being in a constant state of stress is only going to make it harder for you to keep from overeating and it will also make you crave the kinds of foods that are bad for you. Not to worry, though!

With regular yoga practice and physical exercise as a part of your daily routine it will be easy for you to kick your stress habit to the curb and be the healthiest version of yourself that you can be.

Chapter 3: 15 Yoga Poses for Weight Loss

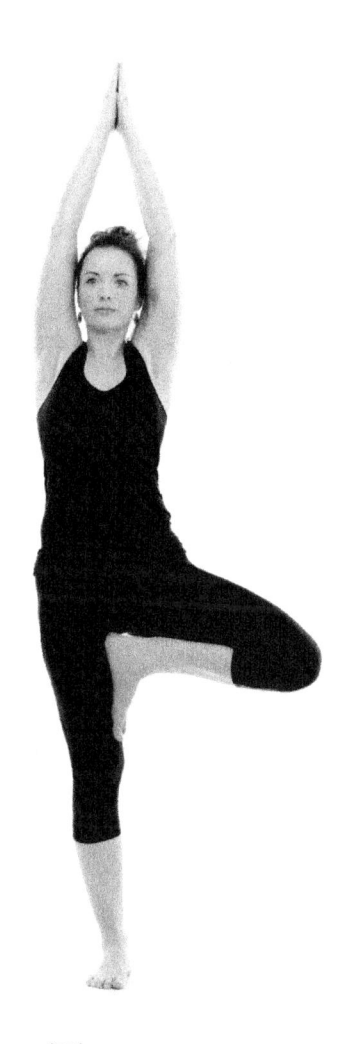

Tree Pose

Step 1: First, stand in Mountain pose and begin to shift your weight a little bit onto your left foot. Keep the inside of the foot firm on the floor and bend the right knee. Slowly reach down and grab your right ankle with your right hand.

Step 2: Pull your right foot up and place it against your inner left thigh as high as you can to where it feels comfortable. Your goal should eventually be to press your right heel into your left groin completely flat with your toes pressing down toward the floor. Keep your pelvic bone directly over your left foot.

Step 3: Visualize lengthening your tailbone, getting it as long as you can. Press your right foot into your inner thigh and then place your hands in the prayer position in front of you, looking straight ahead.

If you don't want to put your hands in prayer position you can place them on your hips or at your sides.

Stay in this position for 1 minute, breathing evenly.

Targets: core and sides of abs, as well as stabilizing leg muscles

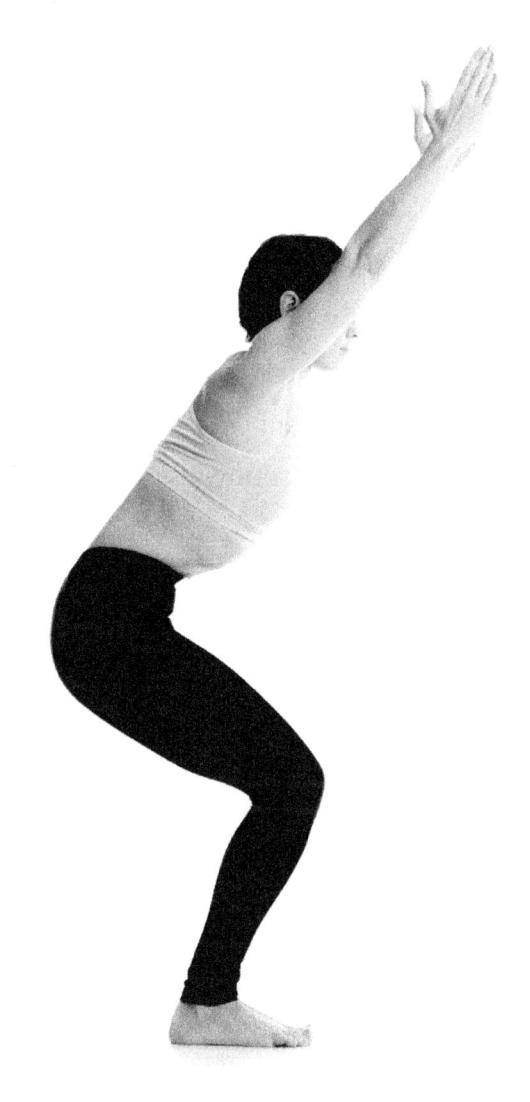

Chair Pose

Step 1: Begin in Mountain pose. As you inhale, bring your arms perpendicular to the ground. You can clasp your hands together or you can keep your arms parallel, palms inward—whatever is most comfortable.

Step 2: As you exhale, bend the knees and bring your thighs as parallel to the ground as possible. Your knees will be over your feet and torso will be slightly forward above the thighs until you're at a right angle with the tops of your thighs. Press your thighbones down into your heels.

Step 3: Keep your shoulder blades firm and push your tailbone down toward the ground and inward to your pubic bone. Try to keep your lower back elongated.

Stay in this position for 1 minute. Inhale and lift your arms, as you exhale release and bring your body back into Mountain pose.

<u>*Targets:*</u> *butt and thighs*

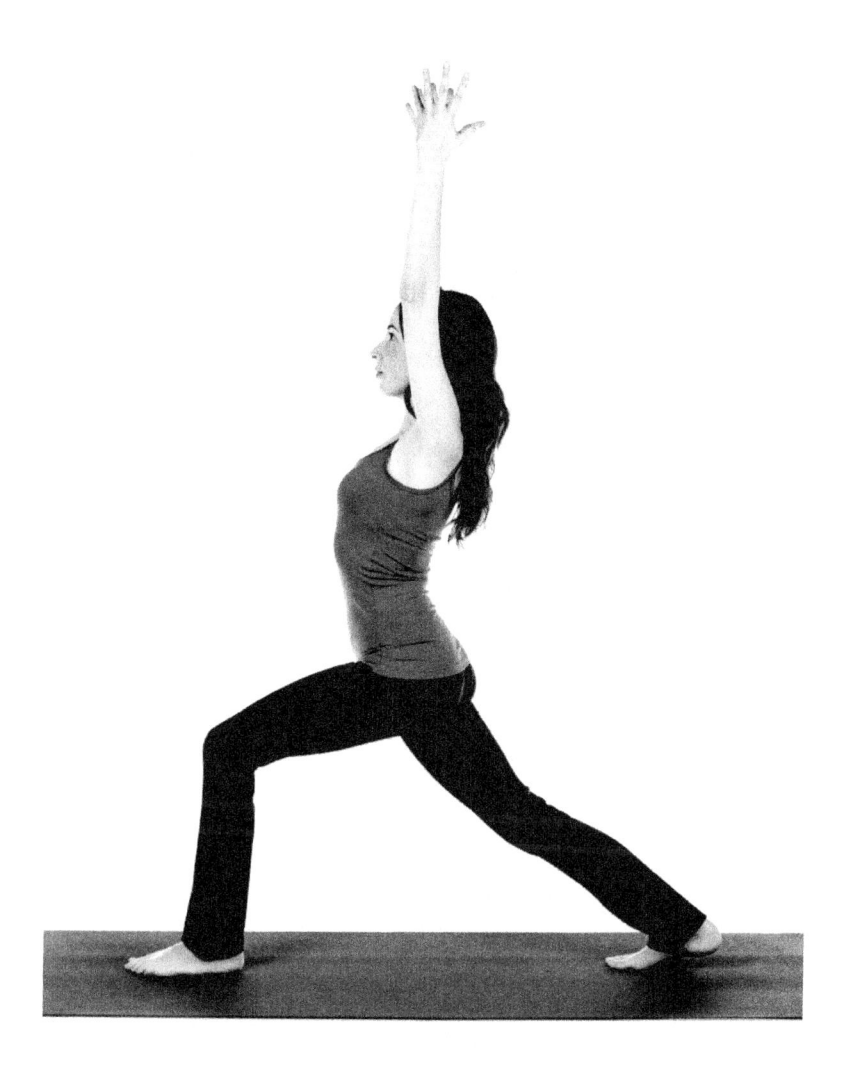

High Lunge Pose

Step 1: Position yourself in the Standing Forward Bend pose and bend your knees slightly. As you inhale, step back with your left foot to the edge of your mat, making sure that the ball of the foot is what's on the floor. You want to be back far enough that your right knee forms a right angle.

Step 2: Now, position your torso over your front right thigh and stretch, making yourself as tall as you can. Loosen your groin region by imagining that your right thigh is melting towards the floor while looking forward. At the same time, keep your left thigh firm and pull it up toward the ceiling while you keep your left knee straight and stretch the left heel down toward the floor.

Step 3: As you exhale, step the right foot back and go into Downward Facing Dog. When you inhale again, step your left foot forward between your hands and repeat the lunge on the opposite leg.

Stay in this position for 1 minute, breathing evenly. Then repeat on the opposite side.

<u>Targets:</u> *abs, arms and glutes*

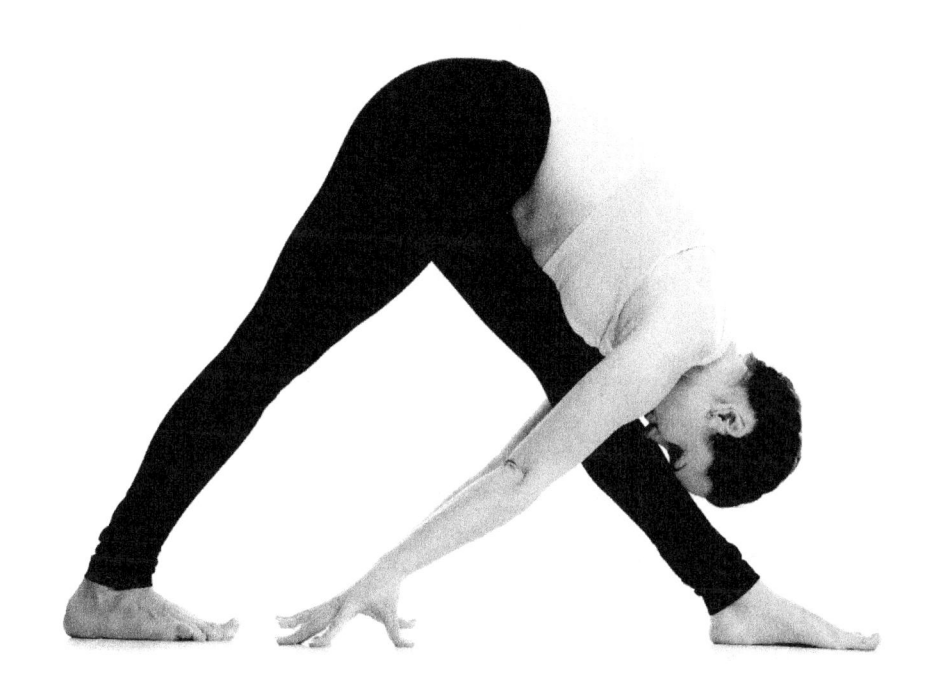

Intense Side Stretch Pose

Step 1: Start off in Mountain Pose. As you exhale, step your feet apart 3-4 feet and rest your hands at your hips. Rotate your left foot inward about 45-60 degrees to your right and place your right foot out at 90 degrees. Be sure to keep your heels in alignment. Keep your thighs firm and push your right thigh outward—the goal is to align your kneecap over your ankle.

Step 2: As you exhale, rotate your torso to your right so that your pelvic bone is square to the edge of the mat. As you point your left hip forward, press your femur bone back to help ground your heel. Visualize pressing a block between your inner thighs and firm your shoulder blades as your lengthen your body down toward the floor. You should be arching your torso slightly back.

Step 3: Exhale again and lean your torso forward over your right leg, stopping when you're parallel to the floor. Now press your fingers onto the floor beside your right foot, stabilizing yourself. If you can't touch the floor then use a block or a chair. Lift the top of your sternum as you press your thighs back and lengthen yourself.

Step 4: Be mindful to keep your front hip soft while continuing to squeeze your outer thighs. The base of your big toe and inner heel should be planted firmly into the floor as you lift your groin and front part of your pelvis.

Step 5: Keep your head and torso parallel to the floor and breathe deeply for 5-10 breaths. If you can do so, start to deepen the stretch by bring your torso even closer to the top of your thigh being mindful not to round your back. Hold for 15-30 seconds and release on the inhale.

Stay in this position for 1 minute, breathing for 5-10 breaths then switch to the opposite leg.

Targets: abs, hamstrings and legs

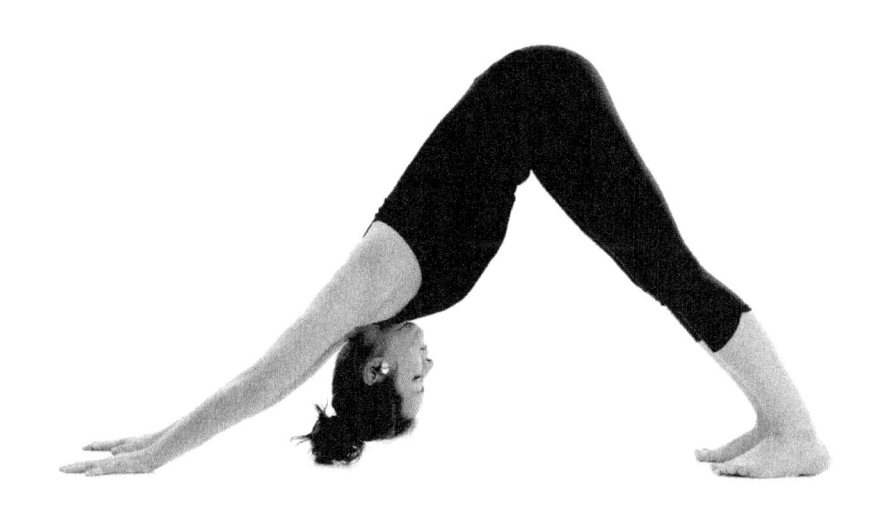

Downward Facing Dog

Step 1: Get on the floor on your hands and knees so that your knees are right below the hips and your hands are slightly in front of your shoulders as you keep your toes pointed under.

Step 2: As you exhale, bring your knees away from the mat and keep a slight bend as you lift your heels away from the mat. Focus on lengthening you tailbone and gently press it toward your pubic bone. Lift your butt high toward the ceiling and bring your ankles into the groin.

Step 3: On another exhale stretch your heels down to the mat and straighten your knees—but don't lock them. Keep your arms firm and press your palms into the mat as you draw your shoulder blades back and stretch them. Keep your head in line with your spine making sure to not let it hang.

Stay in this position for 1 minute, breathing evenly.

<u>*Targets:*</u> *arms, abs and legs*

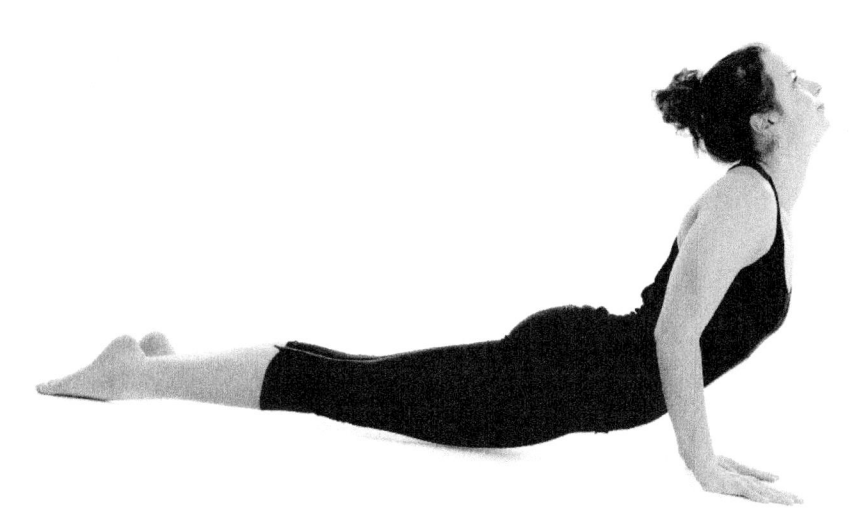

Cobra Pose

Step 1: Lie on your stomach in the floor with your legs out behind you and the tops of your feet touching the floor. Next, place your hands on the floor directly under your shoulders as you press your elbows back and into your sides.

Step 2: Place pressure on the tops of your feet and thighs and pubic bone as you press yourself firmly into the floor. As you inhale, straighten your arms and lift your chest off the floor. Make sure that you don't go so far that you're pubic bone is off the floor.

Step 3: Keep your shoulder blades firm as you "puff" your chest forward, lifting through the top of your sternum. Be mindful not to tighten your lower back. If you notice quite a bit of lower back pain or pressure, feel free to widen the distance between your legs as this should help.

Stay in this pose for 30 seconds as you continue to breathe slowly and evenly. Release on the exhale.

Targets: abs, arms and glutes

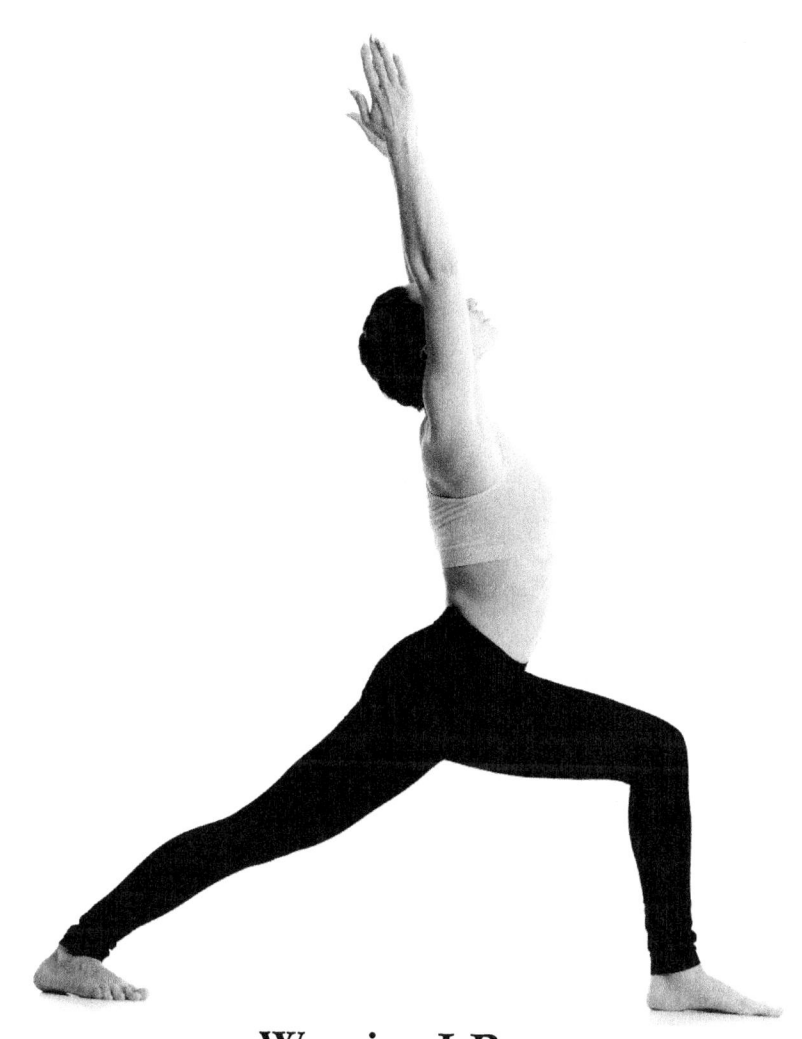

Warrior I Pose

Step 1: Start off in Mountain pose and then exhale as you bring your left foot back behind you 3-4 feet. Now, turn your left foot outward to 45 degrees as you keep your right foot forward.

Step 2: Make sure to keep both of your hips facing forward and parallel to the floor as you bring your shoulders forward as well. Inhale and then raise both arms perpendicular to the floor. Be sure to keep them open and shoulder width apart.

Step 3: Reach up towards your fingertips and face your palms inwards while pulling your shoulders back away from your neck. As you exhale engage your ab muscles and bring your pelvic bone down.

Step 4: Carefully move your right knee forward and align the knee over the heel. Keep breathing and make sure the pressure is located in your right heel and not your toes.

Step 5: Be sure to keep your head neutral by either looking forward or by tilting your head back to look up toward your thumbs.

Stay in this pose for up to 1 minute and then repeat on the opposite side.

Targets: *hips, abs and thighs*

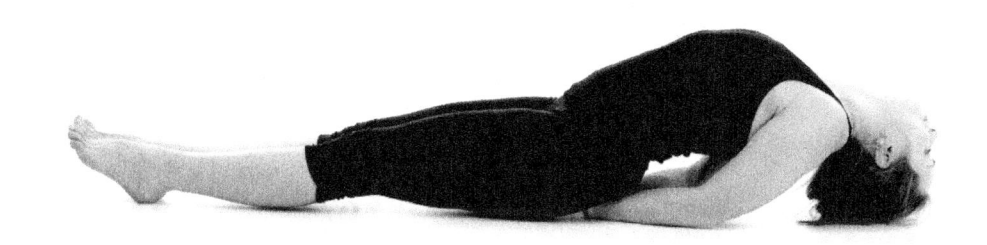

Fish Pose

Step 1: Start out lying on your back on the floor with your knees bent and feet flat on the floor. As you inhale, lift the pelvis off the floor slightly as you slide your hands (palms down) to the base of your butt. Rest your butt on the backs of your hands and keep yourself planted for the duration of the pose, never lifting up off your hands. Keep in mind to tuck the forearms and elbows into the side of your torso.

Step 2: As you inhale, press the forearms and elbows firm against the floor and your shoulder blades into your back. On another inhale, list the upper part of your torso and your head off the floor and then slowly release your head back onto the floor. You should either be resting your head on the back or the crown—it just depends on how high the arch is in your back and how high your chest is lifted. Just be sure to avoid placing a significant amount of weight on your head so you don't hurt your neck.

Step 3: You can either straighten your legs or keep them bent. However, if you choose to straighten them you'll want to be conscious to press out through your heels so that your thighs stay engaged.

Stay in this position for 30 seconds as you inhale and exhale deeply.

<u>*Targets:*</u> *arms, abs, legs and back*

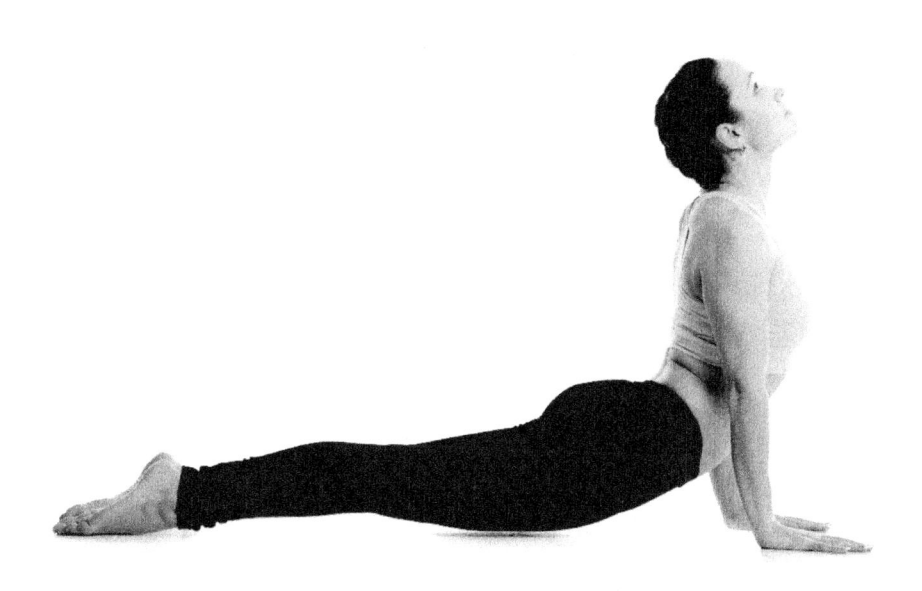

Upward Facing Dog

Step 1: Lie in the floor on your stomach and extend your legs out behind you with the tops of your feet pressed against the floor. Move your forearms perpendicular to the floor and place your palms on the floor on either side of you.

Step 2: As you inhale, press your hands into the floor like you're going to do a push up, straighten the arms as your lift your torso and legs off the floor.

Step 3: Push your tailbone down toward your pubic bone and lift your pubic bone to your belly button. Push your shoulder blade back and lift your chest, but don't puff it out. Be careful not to create tension in your lower back. If this happens you can spread your legs wider to relieve the pressure.

Stay in this pose for up to 1 minute. If you feel like you need to counteract the backbend you can do a Child's pose afterward.

<u>*Targets:*</u> *arms, abs and legs*

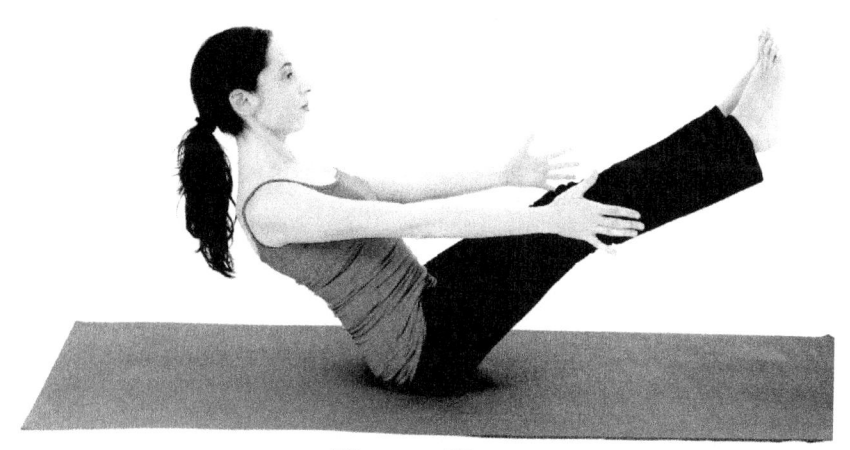

Boat Pose

Step 1: In a sitting position put your knees and feet together with your knees bent. Hold the backs of your knees and focus on lengthening the spine as you lean back slightly making sure not to fold over as you find the edge of your butt bones.

Step 2: Stare straight ahead and as you inhale bring your feet a couple inches off the ground, balancing on your butt, breathing in and out as you find your balance.

Step 3: Stay tall as you gently raise your heels to knee level, keeping your knees bent. If you can complete this easily and you're comfortable then let go of your legs and bring your arms forward as you keep chest broad. If you still feel good and steady you can raise your legs at a diagonal in the air in front of you taking care not to round your back.

Stay in this position for as long as you can, but at least 30 seconds.

Targets: abs and back

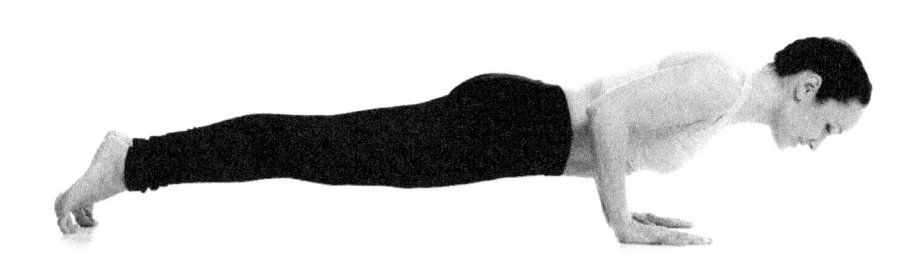

Chaturanga Pose (Four Limbed Staff)

Step 1: Get into Downward Facing Dog and then go into Plank Pose. Keep your shoulder blades firm and your tailbone pulled toward your pubic bone.

Step 2: As you exhale, gently lower the torso and legs just a couple inches parallel to your mat. Be mindful to keep your back properly aligned and straight and keep your pubic bone tucked inward toward the belly button.

Step 3: Make sure to broaden your shoulder blades and keep your elbows close to your sides as you press your fingers into the mat. Left your sternum and head so that you're looking forward.

Stay in this position for up to 30 seconds if you can.

Targets: arms, shoulders, abs and back

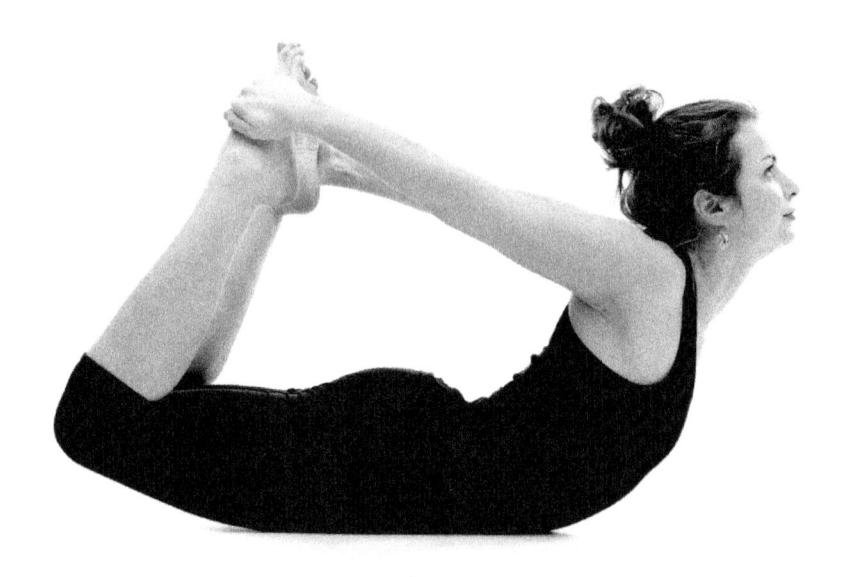

Bow Pose

Step 1: Start off lying on your stomach in the floor with your hands on either side of your torso, palms facing up. If you need to, you can roll up a blanket to provide extra cushioning if it hurts your stomach.

Step 2: As you exhale, bend the knees and bring your heels as close to your butt as you can. While doing this, reach back with both hands and grab onto your ankles. Keep your knees hip width apart for the entire length of the pose.

Step 3: On the inhale, lift your heels away from your butt and thighs away from the floor with a significant amount of strength. By doing this you'll pull the upper torso and your head off of the floor. Soften your back muscles and push your tailbone down into the floor. Focus on lifting your thighs and heels higher into the air and press the shoulder blades firmly into your back in order to open up your heart. Be sure to keep the top of your shoulders away from your ears and look straight ahead.

Please note: this pose makes it somewhat difficult to breathe smoothly and deeply, but keep breathing! Focus on breathing into the back of your torso.

Stay in this position for 30 seconds, focusing on your breathing technique. As you exhale, release yourself gently and lie flat for a couple breaths.

<u>Targets:</u> *back muscles and core*

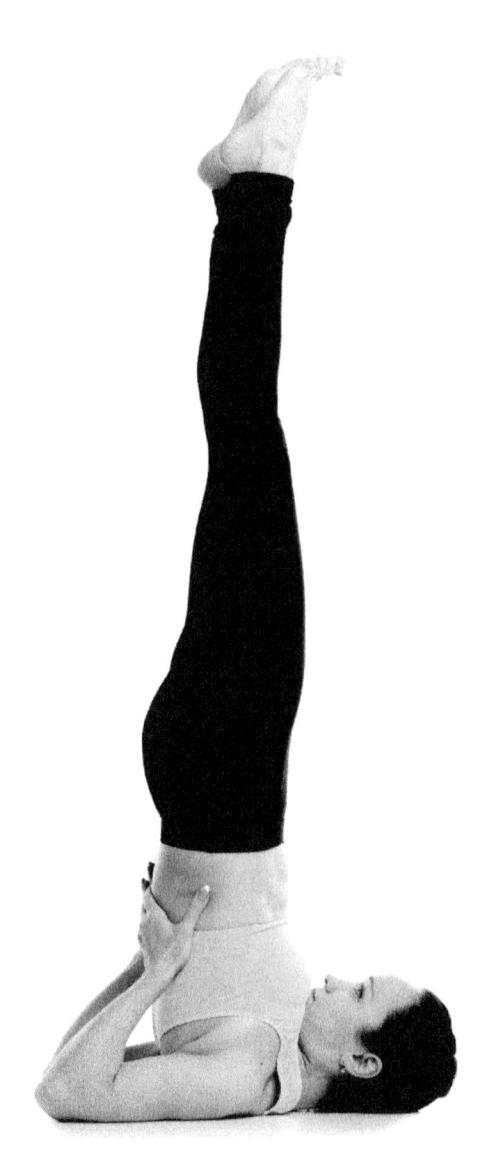

Supported Shoulder Stand

Step 1: First, you'll want to prepare your space. Do so by folding several firm blankets into rectangles stacked on top of each other. You'll want to make them big enough that you have enough room to position yourself into the pose comfortably—

about 1 foot x 2 feet. If you want to you can also put a mat over the blankets so it's easier to grip while in your pose.

Step 2: Now, lay on the blankets with your shoulders being supported and head on the floor as you keep your arms out to your side. Next, bend the knees and put your feet on the floor with your heels in close to your butt. As you exhale, push your arms into the floor and your feet away from the floor as your draw your thigh into your torso.

Step 3: Curl your pelvis and back torso up and away from the floor as you continue to lift yourself and your knees come to your face. Next, position your arms parallel to the edge of your blanket and press your fingers against the floor, thumbs pointing behind you. Bend the elbows and draw them to each other. Your upper arms should be resting against the blanket and palms spread against the back of your torso as your raise your pelvic bone over your shoulders so that you're perpendicular to the floor. Slowly walk your hands toward the floor (up your back) as you focus on keeping your elbows shoulder width.

Step 4: As you inhale, life your knees up to the ceiling and line your thighs up with your torso while you let your heels hang down by butt. Press the tailbone into your pubic bone and squeeze your upper thighs. On another inhale, straighten your knees and press your heels up to the ceiling. When you've fully extended your legs, lift through the balls of your big toes and hold yourself here.

Step 5: Be mindful of your body and soften the places that are tense. However, keep your shoulder blades firm against your back and press your sternum up toward your chin. The forehead should be parallel to the floor and chin perpendicular. In order to strengthen your base you can press the backs of your arms and tops of your shoulders into the blanket for more support. You should be trying to lift the upper part of your spine off the floor and be looking at your chest.

If you're a beginner, stay in this position for about 30 seconds. You can increase this amount my 5-10 seconds each day that you practice until you become more comfortably. Eventually you should be able to hold this pose for several minutes at a time.

Take your time coming out of this pose as you exhale and bend your knees, while rolling your back and torso slowly back onto the floor.

<u>Targets:</u> *arms, abs and glutes*

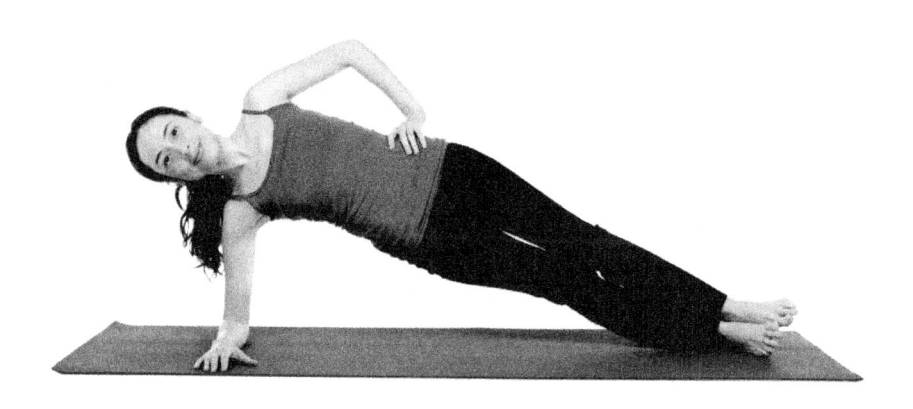

Side Plank Pose

Step 1: Start off in Downward Facing Dog and then shift to the outside of your left foot. Stack the right foot on top of the your left and then place your right hand on your right hip. As you do so, turn your torso to the right and place the majority of your body weight on your left side.

Step 2: You don't want your left hand below your shoulder—keep it slightly in front so that it's at an angle in relation the floor. Straighten your arm by engaging your triceps and then press your index finger into the floor.

Step 3: Keep your shoulder blades firm and pressed into your back as you tighten your thighs and press your heels into the floor. Your entire body should be aligned in a diagonal—from crown to heels.

Step 4: For more of a challenge you can raise your right arm up to the ceiling, parallel to your shoulders as you keep your head in a neutral position or turn to look at the top of your extended hand.

Stay in this position for 30 seconds, breathing evenly and keeping your core muscles engaged. Go into Downward Dog for a few breaths and then repeat on the other side.

<u>*Targets:*</u> *wrists, arms, abs and glutes*

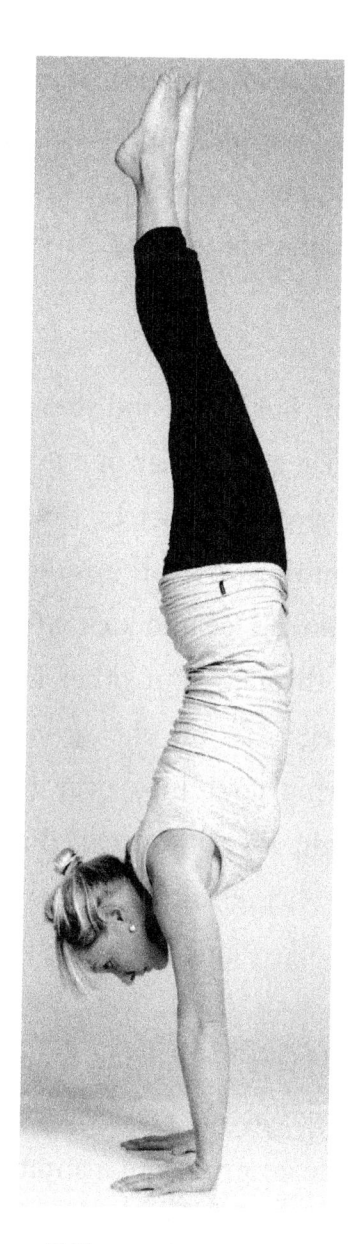

Handstand

Step 1: Start in Downward Facing Dog so that your fingers are a couple of inches away from a wall—shoulder width apart. If you feel like you have tight shoulders you can turn the index fingers out a little, otherwise keep them parallel. Tighten your shoulder blades into your back and pull them to your tailbone while rotating the upper arms out to broaden your shoulder blades. Keep the palms spread and press your index fingers firmly into the floor.

Step 2: Bend one of your knees and step your foot in closer to the wall, while you keep the other one extended through your heel. Get into your pose mindset by doing a few small hops before completely putting yourself upside down. When you're ready, take your extended leg and kick off the floor while at the same time pushing through your other heel to straighten the knee. Once both legs are off the ground, keep your core engaged to help bring your hips over the shoulders. These practice "hops" might be all you can do for now and that's okay—just keep practicing until you feel comfortable and do strengthening poses like Plank to engage your core muscles.

Step 3: However, if you feel strong then go for it. Kick your leg off the ground so that you can bring both legs up onto the wall. If you feel like your groin and armpit areas are tense then the lower back might have a rather deep arch. If you need to lengthen it, draw your ribs into the torso and push your tailbone to your heels while sliding them higher up the wall. Keep your head between your shoulder blades and look out into the center of the room.

As a beginner, try to stay in this pose for at least 15 seconds as you focus on breathing deeply. Keep practicing until you can do this pose for a minute or more. Also note that you should alternate your kicking leg each day.

<u>*Targets:*</u> *wrists, shoulders, arms and core stabilizing muscles*

By practicing these poses you will gain strength in areas that may feel quite weak to you right now. Over time, though, you will begin to feel strong and what was once hard for you will soon become your warm-up.

After you master these poses you might even feel comfortable enough to take a Vinyasa Flow or PowerYoga class!

How Does Yoga Promote Weight Loss?

Many people would say that yoga is much too tame and relaxed of an exercise to provide weight loss benefits. And when you think "yoga" you might not think of cardio. For most forms of yoga that may be true—however, when you look at the practice of PowerYoga then you quickly realize that yoga *can* be even more beneficial than sweating it out on the treadmill at the gym for an hour.

PowerYoga and other vigorous forms of yoga practice offer tremendous cardiovascular and fat burning benefits through their intense breathing techniques and fast paced and challenging movements and flows—just like other forms of aerobic exercise.

But remember: exercising for weight loss isn't just about how many calories you burn, it's also about the muscles and parts of your body you engage. In order to maximize your time and effort spent I would suggest making it a goal to practice yoga at least 5 days a week for a minimum of 60 minutes per day at a rather intense rate of pace.

The weight loss benefits of regular yoga practice don't just show up on the scale. You'll also begin to notice subtle changes in yourself and your thinking patterns. You will be more open to change and have a much greater mind-body connection that will help you overcome bad habits that were previously hard to get rid of.

The habits you develop through yoga are long-term and life changing habits. The difference between changing yourself through yoga and "going on a diet" in the traditional sense of the phrase—is that yoga gives you internal power and motivation: a *reason* for change. When you "go on a diet" it's an external force that you're trying to make yourself go along with, whereas the changes that stem from yoga practice are long-lasting and come from a place of love—for yourself and others.

Tips for Beginners:
- Practice somewhere without mirrors—this lets you focus on how you *feel* and not on how you *look*

- Rest when you're tired—don't push your body to do more than it feels capable of
- On the same note: be mindful of your "comfort zone" and push slightly past that point
- Set a schedule and stick to it—commit to a certain time each day to work on your yoga practice
- Learn to focus on each movement and how every part of your body is feeling and responding to it
- Be patient with your body and talk to yourself lovingly
- Realize that your yoga practice brings you closer to who you really are—inside and out—and by becoming the best version of you, you are inspiring others to do the same

Just because it's *possible* to lose weight through the practice of yoga, it definitely doesn't mean that it's going to be easy. However, as long as you commit to the exercise regimen and take an honest look at your diet in the next chapter, then there won't be anything stopping you from achieving your weight loss goals through yoga.

Chapter 4: Yoga, Food and You

So now that you know all about the different types of yoga and how they can help you lose weight, let's take a look at the other side of the spectrum: your diet. When I use the term 'diet' I don't mean it in the modern sense of the word, which generally translates to mean restriction more than anything else.

This is not what I am referring to at all. No, when I say 'diet' I mean your habitual eating patterns and how we can change those eating patterns to better suit a healthier lifestyle and long-term weight loss success.

If we look at traditional yogic philosophy, their diet was considered one of the most important aspects of their practice. Why? Because if you're not nourishing the tissues and cells of the body with the correct food then you're not going to have proper control over your mind or emotions.

However, there are no specific menus or guides laid out in ancient yogic texts. Patanjali didn't include a chapter in his *Yoga Sutras* about what a typical "yogic diet" should be. Many yoga practitioners focus on Patanjali's 5 yamas for inspiration with their diet—more specifically, Ahimsa (non-violence/non-harming). When it comes to diet, most yogis interpret this to mean that you need to be vegan or vegetarian if you are trying to practice Ahimsa in all aspects of your life.

It all comes down to *your* inner voice—what *you feel* will promote health, longevity, peace and clarity in your own life. This is going to be different for everyone and should be celebrated and respected as an individual's choice of how best to honor his or her own body.

There are plenty of people who try to be vegan or vegetarian, but just don't have good luck with it. They commit to it for years and cling to the hope that this is "how it's supposed to be." But the truth is: not everyone was designed to be compatible with following a vegan or vegetarian diet. Some people feel and operate their best with a little meat in their diet, some a lot. Don't get too hung up on what other people are eating or not eating. Also keep in mind that you should eat to live, not live to eat.

If a type of diet is making you sick and causing you to not function normally then it's not the diet for you—whether it's vegan, vegetarian or omnivore. Listen to your body: it will tell you what it needs.

Maybe you're curious as to what options you have as far as your diet goes. Below I will go over a few different diets and what they consist of. Feel free to experiment and see which one makes you feel best. Maybe it's even a combination of a few different diets. I encourage you to really listen to your body and pick what makes you feel the best—don't feel pressured to fit into any certain label or have a bunch of "rules." Remember: there is one truth, but **many** paths.

Defining Diets

Vegan—a person who does not eat or use animal products.

Diet staples: Almond milk, tofu, beans, nuts/seeds, brown rice, quinoa, nutritional yeast, maple syrup, coconut oil—and of course lots of fruits and veggies.

Avoids: Meat, anything made of animal by-product (butter, eggs, dairy, leather, fur, honey, etc.)

Vegetarian—a person who does not eat meat. Depending on the person, this may or may not include dairy or eggs.

Ovo-Vegetarian—a person who does not eat meat, but does eat eggs.

Lacto-Vegetarian—a person who does not eat meat, but does eat dairy.

Ovo-Lacto-Vegetarian —a person who does not eat meat, but does eat eggs and dairy.

Diet staples: Plant-based oils, eggs (depending on whether or not you're ovo-vegetarian), nuts/seeds, legumes, whole grains and again—lots of fruits and veggies.

Avoids: Meat, eggs & dairy (depending on the type of vegetarian), gelatin.

Omnivore —a person that eats both plants and animals.

Diet staples: meat, eggs, fish, dairy, whole grains, legumes, fruits and vegetables.

Avoids: Not much of anything, unless the person has a particular allergy—this is the least restrictive type of diet on the list.

Pescatarian —a person that doesn't eat meat, but does eat fish.

Diet staples: fish, shellfish, nuts/seeds, legumes, whole grains, fruits and vegetables.

Avoids: Meat from land animals and depending on how strict their diet is they may choose to refrain from any animal-based products.

Sattvic/Yogic—a person that eats foods based on the sattva qualities (energetic, clean, conscious, honest, seasonal, etc.). This is sometimes referred to as the traditional Yogic Diet.

Diet staples: legumes, whole grains, tofu, plant-based oils, nuts/seeds, natural sugars, sweet spices, all fruits and vegetables (but no garlic or onions).

Avoids: Meat and fish, eggs, processed foods, animal fats, garlic/onion, anything spicy, white flour/sugar, canned foods, microwaved food, GMO's.

Plant-based—a person that eats mostly fruits, vegetables, whole grains, legumes. Different from vegetarian in the sense that people who follow plant-based diets do eat meat on occasion.

Diet staples: Meat (sparingly), whole grains, legumes, plant-based oils, almond milk (or other non-dairy milk), nuts/seeds, lots of fruits and vegetables.

<u>Avoids:</u> Excessive amounts of meat, dairy products, eggs, white flour/sugar.

Raw Food—a person that eats only raw, living foods. This includes vegetables, fruits, leafy greens and nuts and seeds. These foods are never cooked.

<u>Diet staples:</u> All raw fruits and vegetables (they avoid tubers), dehydrated fruits and vegetables, raw nuts/seeds, freshly pressed vegetable juices.

<u>Avoids:</u> Anything cooked. This would be the most restrictive diet on the list.

I think that you'll find the longer you practice yoga, the more in tune you will become to how your body feels after you consume certain types of foods. If you eat something that upsets your digestion and makes it harder for you to perform certain poses or focus, then chances are you'll learn to avoid it.

Your goal here should be to eat for clarity and nourishment of your body on all levels. There should be no pressure to conform to any certain label and I actually encourage you to refrain from labeling yourself as any one thing.

Please keep in mind, though, that our body's needs *do* change: just because you didn't do well on a vegan or vegetarian diet 10 years ago doesn't mean you wouldn't now. It's all about experimentation and being willing to change your diet to meet the needs of your body *right now*.

Yoga & Digestion

If you truly focus on how your diet affects your yoga practice then you'll also want to think about the role that digestion plays as well.

It's so important, in fact, that many instructors suggest waiting 3-4 hours after eating a meal to practice yoga. Otherwise your body will be putting all of its energy into digesting your meal and you won't have any to expend during your practice. This is why you need to fuel your body with foods that promote lightness and vibrancy.

This is also why many people who are serious about their yoga practice follow the Sattvic, or Yogic, Diet. Sattvic foods are those that provide prana (or life force) for our bodies and are grown harmoniously within nature. The Sattvic Diet also believes that the foods we eat should be prepared with positive intentions and love, which is another reason to eat at home more often.

Sattva Approved Foods
- Vegetables, but avoid garlic and onion
- Fruits
- Nuts and seeds (raw)
- Legumes
- Rice, wheat and oats
- Plant-based oils (olive, sunflower, sesame)
- Maple syrup, molasses, raw sugar
- Spices like cardamom, cinnamon, basil, mint, turmeric, cumin, ginger and fennel

Foods You Should Avoid
- Meat, including eggs
- Processed food
- Margarine or animal fat
- Anything fried
- Canned food, except those canned at home
- Anything spicy
- White sugar and flour
- Overly cooked food
- Anything microwaved
- GMO's

Eating in this manner ensures that your mind, body and spirit are all in tune with each other and your energy levels are stable and digestion is optimal.

By keeping your digestive needs in mind when eating certain foods you're less likely to cause upset in your body and more likely to feel your best at all times. If you know that certain foods don't digest properly for you—then avoid them!

I personally cannot consume dairy or wheat products. They just don't serve my body well and I end up having all kinds of issues after eating foods containing these ingredients. For me, it's just not worth feeling bad for a moment of pleasure. And honestly, foods like that aren't pleasurable to me any longer because I've learned to associate them with the harmful and negative effects they have on my body.

When you start caring about your body and what you put in it, your body can start caring for you as well—the way that it was meant to. Most of us have never experienced what true health feels like so we don't know what we're missing out on. I used to binge on pizza and ice cream and chips and feel like crap afterward, but I just told myself that that was normal. And for a lot of people that is normal behavior, but only because they don't know what the alternative could be.

If you've ever woken up feeling excited and light and happy to take on the day then you know what I'm talking about. If you eat in such a way that you wake up feeling sick or groggy or in pain almost every morning, then something needs to change.

I'm not saying these things to make you feel bad about your choices, I'm saying them to you because I care and I want you to feel what true health feels like. That should be your goal: not a number on the scale.

I promise if you invest a month to really focus on your body's needs and taking care of it to help it run its best, you won't ever want to go back to your old way of living—you'll feel too good to turn around and slip back into your old eating habits.

It helps if you also get an accountability partner—maybe a friend or family member or even your spouse to join you on your journey.

When you surround yourself with likeminded people it makes it much easier to stay on track and feel good about what you're doing. Don't worry, though: if you don't have an accountability partner it's not the end of the world, it will just take more work on your part to keep yourself on track, especially if you have family members who frown upon whatever you're doing.

Have no doubt: there will be plenty of people in your life (whether they're people you know, or strangers) who will have an opinion about the different choices you're making in regards to your health. Most of the opinions will be negative, unfortunately, but just know that those opinions are coming from a place of misunderstanding and negativity.

The human race is a pack and when someone strays from the pack and does something that is considered "different" or "weird" it tends to make others feel threatened—especially if these people are uninformed about the choices you're making. It causes them to feel uneasy with themselves, like they're doing something wrong. And believe me, people don't like to be made to feel that way.

If people have negative opinions or thoughts about what you're doing and the changes you're making in your life, simply brush it off. You know your body best and the needs that you have— politely move along and keep at it.

These same people who are trying to scare you away from your new lifestyle are going to be the same ones that, in a month from now, will want to know what you're doing because you look fantastic. All you can do is smile and spread your light and continue on your path of healing and change.

Chapter 5: Mindful Eating

Mindfulness, as a broad term, is simply the ability to focus on the present moment and I'm sure you're aware that through practicing yoga regularly you can begin to develop this habit and be stronger in this area.

In this chapter we're going to focus on mindful eating. Mindful eating goes beyond your diet to focus on the *entire* eating experience and the nourishment of your body through the proper foods.

Based on the definition you might assume that this is an easy thing—to focus on the experience of eating, but with the number of distractions we have in our lives today it's much more difficult than it should be.

Our culture has made eating such a production that, to eat mindfully, can sometimes appear as though you're being rude. Eating has become a powerful and dominant form of social interaction. When we go out to eat with friends or family we are expected to participate in the busy conversation and excitement of whatever else is going on that our thoughts are usually not on our food and what we are putting into our bodies. And heaven forbid if we decline the offer to go out to eat with them.

Not to mention, there are televisions everywhere (at restaurants, in every room of the house), smart phones out, books and newspapers to read, mail, homework, a work project, computers—all of this adds up to major distraction when you're eating at the same time.

My advice to you would be: stop it. Cut out all of these distractions and simply focus on your meal and the sensations you get from eating your food. Be mindful of each and every bite—the taste, texture, smells—engage all of your senses in the eating experience. Consciously chew every single bite until it's the consistency of apple sauce (this ensures proper digestion).

If you feel like it's too difficult for you to be mindful at every meal throughout the day then start out small. Be mindful of **one** meal a day, or even a snack and see how it feels. How does the experience change for you?

At first you might feel like it's a tremendous waste of your time to eat this way. After all, we all want to view ourselves as these masterful multi-taskers who should be able to do several different things all at once. Not to mention we view ourselves as being so busy that we can't even make time to cook for ourselves or our families. However, if you give yourself time to adjust to the experience and increase the amount of time you practice mindful eating each day then you will begin to notice great benefits from it.

By practicing mindful eating you will start to eat less because you will be in tune to your body's internal cues that tell you when you're hungry and when you're full. Often if we're distracted we end up overeating at each meal because we don't notice our body's cue to stop. It can be quite subtle and if you're not listening to your body or consciously checking in with yourself every few minutes then you'll completely miss it.

I use the 80% rule when eating, and being mindful helps to ensure that I'm successful with it. The 80% rule comes from the Okinawan culture. Its originations are from the ancient Confucian teaching 'Hara hachibu'—which translates to 'eat until you are eight parts full (out of ten)', hence the 80% rule.

As a result, if you're overweight and begin practicing the 80% rule you're going to lose weight. If you're at a healthy bodyweight then following this rule will help you maintain your weight with very little effort. If you look at the Okinawans in Japan you'll actually see that their average BMI of adults age 60 and over is much healthier than that of the United States. It's also worth noting that they have the highest population of people over the age of 100—more so than any other culture in the world.

So not only is being mindful while eating great for weight loss and increasing the longevity of your life, but it also offers a more peaceful eating experience overall and helps to foster more gratitude in all aspects of your life. The world we live in is incredibly fast-paced—we eat on the go, at fast food restaurants, in our cars, at our desks—none of this is conducive to a positive eating experience.

When we eat fast food it literally has the word 'fast' in the title. Do you think you're going to sit down and savor every single bite, being conscious of the taste, texture and smell? No. You're not going to want to, either because if you did you probably wouldn't want to keep eating it. It's no secret that the quality of fast food is not the same as eating a crisp, refreshing organic salad from the salad bar at Whole Foods or a thoughtfully prepared meal made at home from scratch with love and positive intention.

All food has energy and the more you're aware of where your food comes from the better you can direct the right types of energy into your body for the best eating experience.

Yoga and mindfulness create an awareness inside of you that makes you want to take care of yourself and do the best for your body that you possibly can. In turn, you also want to take care of and respect other living things. This is why most people who practice Ahimsa refrain from eating animals—they don't want to contribute to the unnecessarily inhumane treatment of animals.

However, as I stated in the previous chapter there are different diets that work for different people. If you're a person who chooses to eat animals, be conscious of your decision and vow to make more of an effort to eat locally sourced animals that are treated humanely through the duration of their life and death and respected for their sacrifice.

How to Be a More Mindful Eater

- *Respect and Honor Your Food—*
  Breathe deeply before digging in and say a simple prayer or expression of gratitude for the meal that's in front of you. When you take the time to consciously give thanks for the food you're about to eat, it nourishes and fosters gratitude for all things in your life.
- *Try a silent meal—*
  If you live alone this should be somewhat easier than those with families, but I encourage everyone to eat in

silence for at least the first 20 minutes of your meal. No TV, no phone, no talking—just focus on the meal and your eating experience. You don't have to do this for every meal, but at least a few nights a week I would suggest it.

- *Serve yourself a smaller portion—*
Being more mindful of your portion sizes and eating in moderation it makes it much easier to keep yourself from overeating. Know that there will always be other opportunities for you to eat and that if you're still truly hungry after eating what's on your plate you can always go back for some more.

- *Don't skip meals—*
When you don't give your body an eating schedule it's harder to stay on track with your dietary goals and being a mindful eater. When hunger strikes there's not much time to prepare if you continually ignore the signs from your body that it needs to eat. Doing this can cause you to simply scarf down whatever is in sight and lead to definite overeating. Be prepared by keeping a healthy snack with you at all times or in your car for these emergency situations so that you don't eat out of desperation.

- *Focus on all your senses—*
As you eat, make it a pleasurable experience. If you find it comforting to eat in dim light, put some candles out

and sit somewhere that's most comfortable to you. You can even put on some light and relaxing music. Also be mindful of the taste, smell, texture and color of everything you're eating. As you begin to practice being more mindful about the taste of your food and how it makes you feel you might notice that your tastes change. You may no longer crave junk food or heavy foods, but instead you might enjoy crisp salads and juicy fruits more.

- *Try going vegetarian once a week—or even one meal a day—*
  If you're the type of person who doesn't feel your best on a completely vegan or vegetarian diet, try having one meal a week as such. This helps out the environment drastically and also boosts your health since you're cutting out some extra meat and increasing your veggies.
- *Eat slowly—*
  This one might seem like a no-brainer, but you might actually be eating much faster than you think. I know that when I started practicing mindful eating I became so much more aware of how hurried and rushed I had felt before while eating my meals—so much so that sometimes I wouldn't even sit down. Give yourself permission to relax and enjoy your meal slowly, savoring each bite and giving thanks as you do.

It might seem somewhat strange to eat this way at first, but as you practice yoga and being more mindful during your practice, it is only natural for it to flow over into the other aspects of your daily routine.

Mindful Meditation to Beat Cravings

If you're someone that tends to have a hard time battling food cravings, then you're not alone. A lot of us are triggered to eat foods that are bad for us based on stress, depression, anger, sadness or even addiction.

If you find that it's hard for you to just simply make the choice to stop eating foods that you don't want to eat any longer then I encourage you to start using a meditation technique developed by Dr. Jamie Zimmerman.

Using the acronym STOP, you will learn how to handle your food cravings by being aware and intentional about whatever action you choose to take.

Step 1: *S* = *Stop*. Stop whatever you are doing and just take a minute.

Step 2: *T = Three deep breaths.* Breathe deeply and focus on your breaths.

Step 3: *O = Observe.* What triggered this craving? What will happen if you act on it? How will you feel afterward?

Step 4: *P = Proceed.* Move on from the craving. Shift your focus to something else that will distract you until the craving subsides. Get outside and go for a walk or write in your journal.

Mindful eating is one of the most effective habits you can master in order to get control over your eating patterns and your battle with the scale. It's not going to solve all of your problems overnight, but with long-term use, the practice of mindful eating will help you effortlessly shed the weight you're wanting to get rid of and help shape you into the best version of yourself.

Chapter 6: Developing Healthy Habits to Lose Weight Faster

In this chapter we're going to go over a simple goal setting technique to help you stay focused throughout your yoga weight loss journey and get the most out of the experience.

Setting Weight Loss Goals

The ultimate goal you should keep in mind when using yoga practice to help you on your weight loss journey is *how you feel*.

Yes, it's a good idea to weigh yourself, especially at the start of your journey so that you'll be able to look back and see how far you've come. However, most people (women especially), tend to get caught up in this ideal number or goal weight that they want to be at. And there's nothing wrong with having an idea in your mind of where you want to be: that's what goals are. The problem, though, lies in the fact that we usually aren't flexible with these goals.

We tend to take an all or nothing approach and beat ourselves up when things don't go exactly as we think they should or we don't lose as much weight in a week as we want to. Somehow this equates to failure in our minds and tends to derail us from any progress that we've actually made.

For me, as a teenager and college student, when I would diet and attempt to lose weight I would weigh myself constantly. At least once a day, but many days it would be several times a day! This is a ridiculous way to live and it's not conducive to your long-term weight loss and health goals. There is no reason to weigh yourself more than twice a month. In fact, if it were up to me, everyone would get rid of their scales and focus on the habits they're creating and how they *feel*.

Who cares if you're counting calories and losing 2 lbs. a week if you're angry and miserable the entire time? Yes, you're seeing results fast, but you're probably going to feel starved after a few weeks and end up bingeing on all the calories and foods you've been "missing out on."

Ultimately, you should be creating a lifestyle that you enjoy and a health routine that you actually get excited about each day. If you're not having fun, then you aren't living. Yeah, it's great to be skinny, but if you're not happy or healthy then what's the point?

You might be asking why you should even care about setting a weight loss goal? If you have an idea in your mind of where you want to be, isn't that enough? No, it's not. The key is to **write down** your goals. People who write down their goals accomplish significantly more throughout their lives than people who don't. It's not enough to just have an idea of where you want to go in your life; you want to be specific so that the Universe can provide for you.

So now that we know the 'why' of goal setting, let's get to the 'how.'

How to Set a Weight Loss Goal

Step 1: Write down everything you want to improve in your life that has to do with your health. This could be how you want to look physically, certain things you'd like to be able to do athletically, any pain you'd like to get rid of, bad eating habits you want to break, a certain clothing item you want to fit into—whatever they are, write them down. Be specific.

Step 2: Next, create a timeline for each of these goals—when you want to accomplish each of them by.

Step 3: Pick the one that's *most important* to you and write a paragraph about it—visualize and be specific about how it will feel when you've successfully reached this goal and why it will mean so much to you. Phrase it as if it's already happened.

Step 4: Look at your goals every single day. Visualize yourself achieving these goals and focus your mind to help you reach them.

Step 5: Don't let anything get in your way of achieving your goals—not Friday night pizza, a physical injury, negative people, or self-doubt. You are bigger than your fears and you can accomplish whatever you put your mind to. You can truly achieve anything you want in life.

Goal Setting Tips & Tricks

- Get a whiteboard and write your daily, weekly and monthly goals on it so that you have them visible
- Create a vision board
- Post your goals all around your house—on the fridge, the bathroom mirror, the ceiling above your bed—keep yourself reminded *why* you're doing this
- Have an accountability partner
- Use positive affirmations

Also, always remember to reward yourself and celebrate all of your successes. If you happen to reach a particular milestone by a certain date then celebrate it! Let's say you meet your 10 lb. weight loss goal in record time—why not reward yourself with something special. Examples of a healthy reward could be a new outfit, a massage, or even just something you've had your eye on for awhile, but couldn't justify purchasing. It's always important to celebrate your victories, no matter how small because they keep you motivated and excited about the positive changes you're making.

My suggestion, though, is to **not** reward yourself with food. Especially if you have a particularly bad food addiction—you're only hurting your progress by slipping back into your old routines and eating habits. It might not seem like a big deal since it's "just this one time," but more often than not it leads to many more meals than just the one.

That's it! You've got all the tools to make it happen. As long as you follow the guidelines I've laid out for you and focus on your goals each day, then you're sure to overcome anything that stands in the way of reaching your weight loss goals. It's not a race, but rather a journey—be mindful during every step of the way and enjoy the process.

Conclusion

Throughout this book we covered quite a bit of information and lots of different techniques and habits that will help you be successful on your yoga weight loss journey.

In order to be the best version of yourself you must incorporate all of these wonderful habits into your life so that you can reach your maximum potential and live the life you were meant to lead. There will be challenges and roadblocks along the way—even naysayers. But as long as you stay focused on your goals then I have no doubt you'll reach them.

Weight loss is just a positive by-product of living the yoga lifestyle. You can go as fast or as slow as you feel is best for you and your body. It's not a race to the finish line—stay positive and enjoy the journey. As long as you never stop pushing forward with your goals and intentions then you will always be a success.